Meditation

Easy techniques to help you
relax and focus

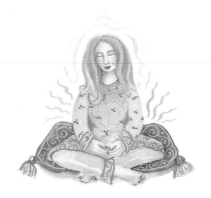

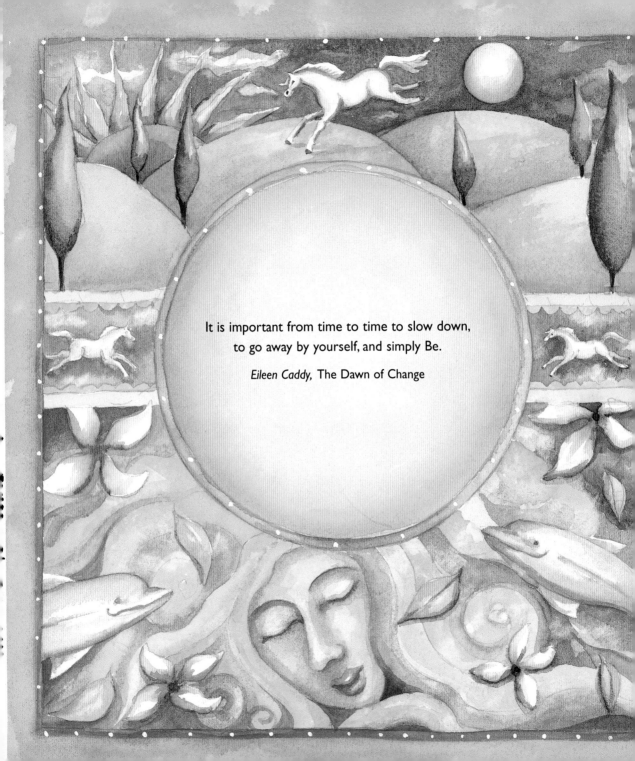

It is important from time to time to slow down,
to go away by yourself, and simply Be.

Eileen Caddy, The Dawn of Change

Meditation

Easy techniques to help you
relax and focus

Jan Purser

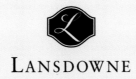

LANSDOWNE

Contents

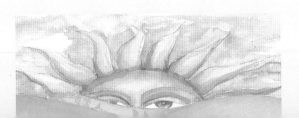

Introduction

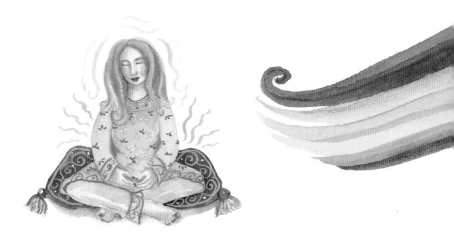

Meditation holds the key to inner contentment and greater peace. To examine the truth of this statement, meditate for 20 minutes daily for one month and compare your contentment, peace and stress levels before and after the month of meditation. It is guaranteed that you will experience more peace and contentment and less stress after practicing meditation.

My version of meditation is one that has developed over many years of practicing and teaching meditation, as well as attending classes, seminars, retreats and workshops related to this inspirational subject. I do not profess that it is the one and only type of meditation to follow. I also make it a point not to push any one particular philosophy or religion in my meditation classes. For me, it is not the details of a specific tradition that count, it is finding a way of bringing the simplest meditative techniques into everyday activities.

It is so important to "live" life, and not simply exist. To do this successfully, it helps to develop awareness or consciousness. Conscious living stands alongside greater inner peace, fulfillment and enlightenment, with meditation providing the path to becoming more conscious and aware.

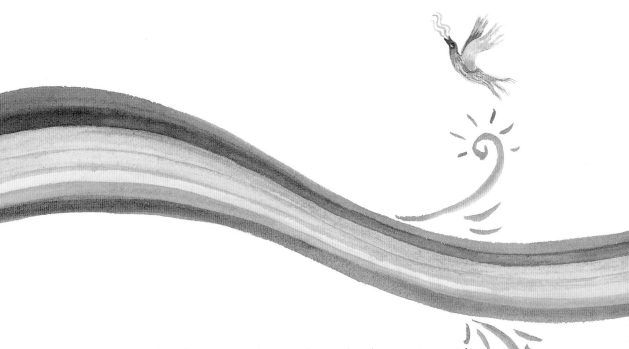

This book, based on my meditation classes, has been written with you in mind, whether you are a little doubtful or whether you are ready to throw yourself into meditation wholeheartedly. There is something here which will appeal to everyone. To gain the most from the book, I recommend you read it from cover to cover and practice the meditation exercises as you go along. You can then flick back to your favorite parts at your leisure and repeat the exercises you enjoyed the most. It could also be useful for you to tape the instructions for the meditation exercises so you can play them back for yourself.

With love and light.

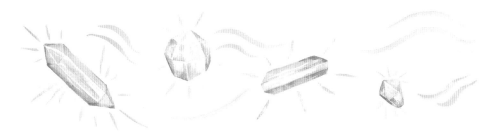

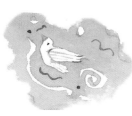

About Meditation

Meditation is very simply the ability to focus on one thing only, allowing thoughts and inner chatter to fall away, leaving a deep feeling of stillness and peace. Some may say it is the path to connecting with your higher self or with a higher consciousness.

In some religions meditation plays a role in the act of praying, giving devotees a sense of being linked to their "god". Many philosophies, such as Buddhism, Taoism and yoga use meditation as an integral part of their faith.

Meditation is not an escape from life or reality. In fact, it is the opposite. When you meditate, you don't cease to hear sound, act responsibly or feel emotions. You become even more alert and focused, and less reactive, but more responsive with emotional issues.

Consider the analogy of a stagnant pool of water which has become murky with fallen leaves, algae build-up and general filth from daily life. There is no fresh water entering the pool to cleanse and refresh it. You cannot see the bottom of the pool and you would never consider swimming in the water for fear of catching some hideous disease that would affect your health. You cannot even see your reflection in the murky depths because all that can be seen is cloudy stagnant water with all kinds of bugs lurking amongst the strands of algae.

Picture a beautiful pool with crystal-clear sparkling water with rays of sunlight dancing across the surface in a display of joyousness. Butterflies and tiny birds dip quickly into the water to take refreshing sips of the cool water. You can see all the way to the bottom of the pool, and when the water is still, you can also see a mirror-perfect image of yourself reflected back from the glassy surface. Fresh water enters the pool daily to create an eternal flow of purity, washing away harmful bacteria, keeping the pool cleansed and renewed.

Now think of your mind on a particularly bad day when your thoughts are in chaos, when you are filled with anger or fear, or with another emotion that creates turmoil. It feels as though there is no way to ease the intensity of your thoughts and the seeming pressure inside your brain from the excessive analyzing and strong emotional activity. This is the murky pool scenario.

Meditation creates space for your mind by stilling the activity and breaking the cycle of "go-nowhere" thoughts. It allows the replenishing of fresh and pure energy to enter your mind and body encouraging clarity, peacefulness and a feeling of well-being – the beautiful pool scenario.

When you meditate and experience this stillness, there is a sense of "coming home". The experience feels as if you have tapped into a part of yourself that you always knew existed but have always seemed unable to reach. It is in fact a "coming home" to the inner or real you – the essence of your soul. This is the part of you that knows no limits to what you can give and feel. It is also the part that knows that, no matter what, everything is perfect as it is.

You often become meditative possibly without realizing it, such as when you are totally focussed on an activity or when you are sitting and gazing out a window without any particular thought in your mind. The times when you are enjoying being by the beach or in the countryside, you can become peaceful simply from being in such surroundings. You may also experience a meditative state when concentrating completely on a physical exercise, such as yoga or dancing, where the sheer effort of performing the movements or steps correctly may still your thoughts.

These activities, naming just a few, are all meditative in some way and show that as human beings we instinctively need to relax our minds to re-energize so that we can carry on with our daily tasks.

Meditation comes in many forms, all of which are beneficial in various ways. And, as the saying goes, the proof of the pudding is in the eating – so put into practice some of the techniques outlined in this book and experience meditation firsthand.

Why should you meditate? When I mention that I teach meditation, people ask me questions like "what is so good about meditating?" and, "do I have to sit cross-legged on the floor and 'om' to meditate?" A common belief is that to start meditating requires changing your entire life. This is not so, although often when you begin to meditate you can feel as though your attitude to your life is changing.

There is a certain amount of mystery surrounding the practice of meditation and yet it is one of the simplest ways of reducing stress in your life. Because it has often been considered a "hippie" kind of thing to do, meditation has, for some people, a negative image.

I always reply to those curious people that they don't have to sit cross-legged on the floor but can meditate anywhere they choose – sitting, standing, walking or lying down. And, no, it doesn't have to involve "om-ing". But more about that later.

There are countless reasons to begin the practice of quietening your mind.

To check if you qualify for needing meditation in your life, use the following handy list. You would reap the benefits of meditation if you:

- feel as though just one more demand on your time may "break the camel's back";
- are often fearful of change or new experiences;
- have inappropriate emotional outbursts or reactions;
- overreact to stressful situations;
- sleep poorly or suffer with insomnia;
- often feel scattered or unfocused in your activities;
- have lost a loved one recently;
- worry that you can't meet the demands of your job or personal life;
- find that your children are too much to handle;
- have trouble communicating peacefully with others;
- feel as though your life is monotonous and routine;
- experience lack of balance between your work and recreation activities;
- are experiencing a relationship breakdown;
- suffer from mild depression;
- feel as though your life is lacking direction or purpose;
- suffer with a chronic illness and are dealing with its associated pain;
- have been diagnosed with a life-threatening illness;
- would like to have more concentration when doing creative tasks;
- would like to feel calm and peaceful more often; or
- wish to improve your performance at a sport or physical activity.

If you relate to two or more items on the list, it is an indication that meditation will improve your life in a way that helps you live in a more peaceful fashion. Just following the basic breathing techniques or pre-meditation relaxation exercises alone will bring some benefits.

Meditation benefits a person on many levels – the physical, mental, emotional and spiritual. Regular daily practice will bring profound changes, while sporadic practice will usually bring benefits for only a short time.

Physically, meditation reduces muscle tension by decreasing the stress response. The deeper breathing that accompanies meditation practice helps to increase circulation of oxygen to the muscles, making them less likely to become tense. High blood pressure will reduce with regular meditation, and as it has been shown that excess stress increases the production of cholesterol, meditation also helps lower high blood cholesterol due to its stress-reducing abilities.

The body's immunity is strengthened as a decrease in stress reduces the "flight or fight" response in the body, minimising the amount of unnecessary adrenaline released. When a person is in a constant state of stress, their body is creating excess adrenaline to cope with the extra demands. Naturopaths call the eventual chronic tiredness associated with this physical response "adrenal exhaustion". One of the tools to help correct this problem is meditation. Meditation also helps you to respond in a conscious way to stressful situations rather than experiencing a "knee-jerk" reaction.

Blood and lymphatic circulation, digestive actions and energy flow are all improved through meditation, due to an improvement to your breathing, movement and the effects of the relaxation response. You will notice when you breathe deeply that your skin will tingle slightly in a very pleasant way, due to the increase in circulation and energy flow through your body. Physical pain, insomnia, tension headaches, anxiety and panic attacks are all reduced by the relaxation response and deeper breathing employed during meditation.

Emotionally, meditation helps you to feel less irritable and "scratchy", particularly when experiencing premenstrual syndrome. It reduces the anger response when confronting difficult situations and helps you to be more objective and peaceful on all levels when communicating with others.

If contending with an emotional trauma, such as loss of a loved one or relationship breakdown, meditation gives your mind the space and stillness needed to detach from the overwhelming emotions and thoughts that occur during such a time.

Mentally, focus, concentration and creativity are increased dramatically with the practice of regular meditation. It opens the energy "channels" to allow for greater creativity and expression for all kinds of artistic endeavors, such as writing, music, painting or dancing.

Some sports people find greater improvement in their performance and skill due to meditation because they are training their minds to remain focused and alert. They use visualization to run faster, hit further, jump higher, or to reach other higher goals.

The improved focus and concentration will be noticeable at the workplace, in business meetings, when completing mind-bending tasks, when undertaking new projects which require a high degree of planning and negotiating, when studying or writing assignments, and when sitting in lectures.

Spiritually, meditation brings about a greater sense of self-awareness and understanding. You will feel connected to all living things and more aware of nature and its importance in your life.

Meditation may also bring to the foreground any issues that are unresolved. For you to feel greater inner peace, issues that have been "swept under the carpet" will have to be dealt with before you can move on. Meditation can be used to help you work out what you need to do with your particular issue. The solution could be as simple as recognizing a better attitude to adopt when dealing with a particular situation or finding a peaceful way of resolving a worrying issue. Whatever the case, you will find lasting peace.

There are many types of meditation which originate in the many philosophies and religions of the world. However, to keep it simple, I like to explain the types of meditation according to the way they are practiced.

Breath-watching meditation

This meditation requires you to focus on the breath entering and leaving your nostrils. The depth of the breath is very important because we do not usually use the full capacity of our lungs when we breathe. To gauge your own breathing, just notice your breath right now and which part of your chest is expanding as you breathe in. Most often our breath is shallow and we only expand the upper part of the chest. Now take several long, slow and deep breaths, being conscious of expanding your entire rib cage and abdomen with the inhalation. On the exhalation, be conscious of forcing all the breath out again before breathing in once more. After a minute or more of doing this deeper breathing, you will already feel more relaxed as the greater flow of oxygen is distributed around your body through your circulatory system.

Visualization meditation

This meditation is very popular. It involves being talked through, or talking yourself through, a scene or scenario while in a meditative state. The idea of the exercise is that you concentrate on the visual picture that you create in your mind – this being the focus for your mind. For stress-relief meditations, the visualization picture is one that creates a feeling of peace and tranquility.

Sportspeople can use visualization meditation to enhance their performance. By picturing themselves excelling at their sport to achieve their goals, they can help promote their confidence and manifest the physical reality of the feat. This principal can also be applied to those wanting to make positive changes in their life. I am sorry to say, this may not apply to winning the lottery if such a win isn't your destiny. However, it can be used to create an abundant outlook that may attract better work opportunities and the means to improve your life in general.

Mantra meditation

The use of a mantra in meditation involves the repetition, out loud or in your head, of particular words which have spiritual significance. "Om" is perhaps the most well-known mantra. It is almost sung, rather than spoken, in such a fashion as to create a humming sound in the ears and a vibrating feeling in the throat, chest and abdomen. The feeling it creates within the body is extremely comforting and helps the mind to quieten and focus.

Music meditation

This meditation is perfect for true music lovers or aficionados, or those who find it difficult to use other meditation methods. As the name suggests, music is the focal point with melodic and peaceful music being the best type of music to use for this exercise.

Walking meditation

Walking meditation doesn't require much space to be performed. For this type of meditation great strides are not usually taken, but little steps. The feet are placed slowly and consciously onto the ground with each step. Particular note is taken of the physical feelings experienced within the foot with each step. It is a very meditative exercise and the focus is in walking slowly and truly concentrating on the placement of the feet.

Object focus meditation

Object focus meditation is where you focus on an object with your eyes open while in a meditative state. Firstly prepare for meditation and then use the object as the focus for your mind. Gaze at the object with soft focus and simply study the object's shape, texture and color and then imagine its smell and feel if applicable. Use objects like a candle, a flower, logs in a fireplace, the ocean, a tree or goldfish. Any object that brings about a recognition of beauty or nature can be used. Obviously, anything moving too quickly or in a distracting fashion is not appropriate.

Posture is very important during meditation and "slumping" should be avoided. You should not feel overly comfortable, as in a lounge chair, as you don't want to fall asleep. In all positions, keeping an extended spine is good practice. Imagine you are being pulled up by the head and feel your spine extending to its maximum length. It may feel a little odd at first, but with practice it will begin to feel comfortable. You can hold your thumbs and forefingers together in the traditional meditation pose if you like. This acts as a signal to your mind that you are now entering a meditation. It also acts energistically – the flow of energy through the energy pathways in your body will be continuous. Here are some suggestions for meditating in the following positions.

Sitting cross-legged

When sitting in this position, it is helpful to sit with your bottom on a high cushion, folded blanket, a couple of pillows, or a few folded towels to place the level of your hips a little higher than your knees. This helps to prevent a feeling of "pins and needles" in your legs from lack of circulation. You will have to concentrate on your posture in this position and make sure you do not slouch your shoulders. You may have to check in every now and then during the meditation to adjust your posture. Your hands can be positioned on your knees or in your lap.

Sitting in a chair

Choose a straight-backed chair which is not so comfortable that you feel like falling asleep and which supports your back well. If you find your back becomes sore or tired during meditation, place a cushion at the small of your back to give you more support. A dining or office chair is a good choice here. Place your feet flat on the floor and your hands softly in your lap or on your knees. Be conscious of keeping your spine lengthened and your shoulders from slouching.

Sitting on the floor

If you are unable to sit cross-legged or find it too uncomfortable, sit on a cushion, pillow or blanket on the floor with your legs out in front of you. Make sure your back is supported by a wall or door. It is a little difficult to sit in this fashion without some support for your back. You may want to place a pillow behind your back for extra support. Place your hands softly in your lap.

Lying down

This is not the best position for meditation as you may drift off into sleep rather than into a meditative state. However, if you choose to lie down, use a firm surface with a small cushion for your head. Lying on the floor is ideal as the floor surface is quite hard and is less likely to make you feel sleepy. While lying down, extend your toes and head as far in opposite directions as you can to straighten your spine. Lay with your arms by your sides with your palms facing upwards. Those people who are able to sleep anywhere without a problem should choose a sitting posture for meditation.

Meditation stool

This specially designed stool is usually made from timber with a firm sitting platform that is only about 10–12 inches (25 cm) or so off the floor. It is perfect for meditation as the sitting platform is at a slight angle to encourage you to sit with good posture. You actually kneel on the floor and then place the stool behind you above your lower legs before you sit down. For more comfort you can place a soft blanket under your legs. As it is usually impossible to fall asleep on the meditation stool it is a good choice for when you are tired or if you tend to fall asleep easily during meditation.

First Steps in Meditation

THE BASIC MEDITATION METHOD

As I tell my classes, the method of meditation is very simple – it just takes a little practice and the observance of the following fundamental basics:

1 Focus on something – breath, object, mantra or music (see *The types of meditation*).

2 Gently push all thoughts aside (see *Taming thoughts*).

3 Let go the expectations of what you think should happen in the meditation, and allow yourself to simply "be" in the meditation. Whatever happens is perfect for that time and place.

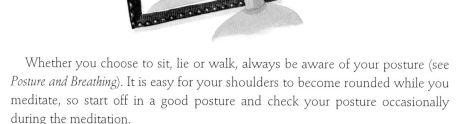

Whether you choose to sit, lie or walk, always be aware of your posture (see *Posture and Breathing*). It is easy for your shoulders to become rounded while you meditate, so start off in a good posture and check your posture occasionally during the meditation.

Before you begin to meditate, do the simple relaxation exercise outlined opposite. It is a good idea to do this first and then follow with the white lighting exercise (see *Self-Protection*).

How to start your relaxation exercise

To prepare yourself for meditation, learn to relax by doing the following:

1 Position yourself for meditation and when ready, take four long, slow, deep breaths, allowing the breath to travel to any areas in your body where you sense tension or tightness. Imagine that breath dissolving the tension into nothingness.

2 Put your legs out directly in front of you, point your toes and then tighten the muscles along the fronts and backs of your legs all the way to your buttocks. Hold the muscles tightly for 20 seconds and then allow them to relax.

3 Tighten the muscles in your stomach and buttocks at the same time. Hold them firmly for 20 seconds and then allow them to soften and relax.

4 Squeeze your shoulder blades together, pushing your elbows behind your body and feeling the tension in the middle of your upper back while expanding your chest. Hold for 20 seconds and then allow your back to relax.

5 Put your arms out directly in front of you, make hard fists with your hands and tighten the muscles all the way up your arms into your shoulders. Push your arms away from your body while you round your shoulders a little until you feel a stretch along your upper back. Hold for 20 seconds and then allow your arms to relax, placing your hands back into your lap or by your sides.

6 Shrug your shoulders as high as you can. Rotate them forward slowly three times and then backward three times. Let them drop softly into a comfortable position.

7 Tilt your head to the left, allowing the weight of your head to increase the stretch along the right side of your neck a little. Hold for 10–20 seconds.

8 Tilt your head to the right side, again allowing the weight of your head to increase the stretch along the left side of your neck. Hold for 10–20 seconds, then straighten your head.

9 Frown, squeeze your eyes shut and purse your lips as hard as you can and then hold for 10 seconds. Allow your facial muscles to soften and relax.

10 Take three more long, slow, deep breaths and imagine the breath dissolving any residual tension in your body. Feel the difference within your body and the heightened sense of relaxation.

When you meditate, you actually open energy centres within your body, which sometimes makes you vulnerable to the energy around you. At the beginning of each meditation, it is good practice to invoke some form of self-protection, such as the "white lighting" exercise opposite.

I also recommend you use this exercise when you first get out of bed in the morning. It helps you to connect with your higher self. It also helps you to be more balanced when dealing with others throughout the day.

While it is not a compulsory exercise to do, I find it invaluable when beginning a meditation. It helps you to reach a meditative state more quickly because energistically you have intentionally connected with the universal energy (the

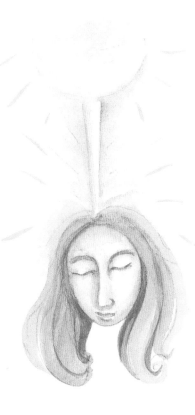

white light). This pure energy offers with it supreme guidance and allows only the highest frequency of energy to come to you while it is being invoked.

If you are feeling a little emotionally unbalanced, or if you have suffered some kind of mental or emotional trauma, this exercise is recommended because it not only helps you to become more centered but it helps you to get in touch with calming and healing energies.

White light used in this fashion is considered to be from the highest possible universal energy source, and deflects any negative energy around you. This negative energy can come from within your own mind, from other people or from places you may visit.

On one occasion, something startled my cat, Bella, who was sitting at my open front door. She was so scared by whatever came near the door that she growled and hissed for many minutes and would not settle or allow anyone to come near her.

I immediately brought white light down around her and around the house and filled the entire house with the light. She settled soon after this and I believe that the act of white lighting helped to dispel any possible dangers to her or myself.

When you "white light" yourself or your surroundings, the white light pushes out and diffuses negative energy around you. This is an exercise you can use when you feel "spooked" about walking down a dark street or in any situation where you feel vulnerable. You can also use this method when you know you have to deal with someone who is difficult. It will help you to maintain a centered composure during the interaction and to see the situation objectively rather than emotionally.

White lighting exercise

Imagine a brilliant white light way above your head. Picture a single beam of pure brightness coming down from this light into the crown, or top, of your head. As you breathe, see that light filling your body slowly, starting with your head and face. The light pours into your body, filling every single cell. Imagine it pouring into your arms right to the very ends of your fingertips. Then see the light filling your torso, buttocks and then legs, pouring into your feet, all the way to the tips of your toes.

Then imagine the light exiting through the bottom of your feet, going deep into the Earth and back up again into your legs. See that light overflowing the top of your head and pouring down around the sides of your body until it forms a cocoon of pure brightness around your entire body, with every part of your body enclosed.

See yourself anchored within this beam of pure white light, which comes from the heavens, to be secured deep in the earth. And feel the protection it offers. It deflects off any negative energy and helps you to retain your own energy without it "leaking" unnecessarily.

Many people comment to me how they believe they can never meditate because they are having a continual and noisy dialogue within their mind. It's true, we imagine all kinds of scenarios, we write the scripts of future encounters and rewrite those from the past. "I could have said this and then they wouldn't have said that...", and so on. We are blessed with intelligence and the ability to analyze and assess. However, the downside of this ability is that our imagination can run away with itself. We can obsess, suffer with "analysis paralysis" and generally not live "in the moment". Our minds are often anywhere but in the moment – usually preferring the past or the future.

Meditation allows us to develop the ability to truly live in the moment – with practice. The trick is to carry this mindfulness and awareness into daily life; this is when you really begin to reap the benefits of meditation.

What to do about those thoughts? Well, the main thing is to expect that they *will* pop up in rapid succession the minute you decide to meditate. Acceptance is part of the cure. Once they begin, you can do a number of things to help slow and eventually quell them:

1 Imagine the thoughts attached to fluffy white clouds drifting across a perfect blue sky and see them float away.

2 See the thoughts as banners going across your "mind screen" – like a computer screen saver – and then moving off the screen altogether.

3 Name the thoughts or categorize them. This can help diffuse them because by naming them you limit their power to distract you. For example, you may categorize a confrontation you have remembered as "anger". If you remember that you are meant to call someone, tell yourself to recall this straight after you cease meditating and then let the thought go, knowing that you will remember later – and you will.

4 Spend some time being the observer of your thoughts. Step onto the "observation platform" and watch the thoughts go by like waves, cars, trains, or boats. By simply observing them like an outsider, you then don't feel the need to become involved with them. They simply come less frequently until finally you realise how still your mind has become.

I always urge my students not to judge how they are "performing" the meditation and not to become annoyed with themselves (and judgmental) if they have trouble stilling their minds. Some days you will slip into stillness like slipping into a pair of your favorite slippers. Other days you will feel as though you have to crawl through a minefield to reach some quiet in your mind. Just accept that each meditation will bring with it a different experience and enjoy the variety it brings. Let's face it, if it was the same time after time, we would probably become bored and lose interest. By having variation it leaves some challenge and diversity in the meditation practice. Below is a simple exercise for letting go of thoughts in your meditation.

Meditation practice – letting go of thoughts

After doing the relaxation and white lighting exercises, allow your breath to return to a normal pace and feel the relaxation continue to flow through your body.

Sit or lie quietly and imagine yourself stepping onto an observation platform just above you and slightly removed from your life. From this position, watch your thoughts come and go. Just observe them – there's no need to develop them into more than what they are. Simply allow the thoughts to waft in and out of your mind like clouds drifting across the sky. If a thought stays a little longer without drifting by easily and seems to need some input, place it in a category, such as anger, worry, love, hurt, lust or resentment. This will diffuse the thought and release it from your mind. Spend a little time now watching the procession of thoughts and see them come less readily and less intensely.

If your mind becomes involved in the thoughts, check if you are on the observation platform and resume your position there if needed.

Meditating at Home and Away

At home

The decision of where to meditate doesn't have to be a difficult one to make. If you intend to meditate on a regular basis at home, may I suggest you keep aside a corner in a quiet room just for this purpose. When you meditate regularly in one spot, you tend to slip into the meditative state more readily, as your mind associates the place with meditation. On an energistic level, you build up a certain type of energy in this one spot. Think of it as a link to the universal energy (see *Self-protection*), by meditating in the same place, you are essentially placing yourself back within the flow of this energy.

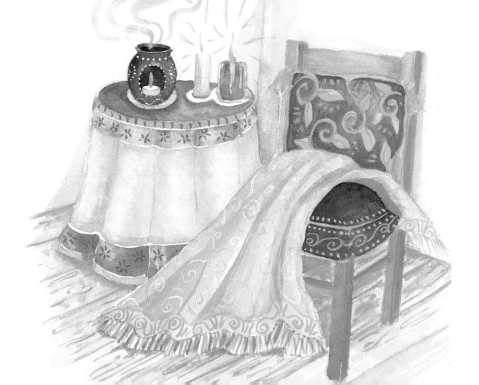

Away from home

You can meditate anywhere you choose. For the most exceptionally challenging meditations, some people meditate in noisy public places, such as major train stations or next to public thoroughfares. They do this to increase their ability to become detached from outside disturbances. If you can meditate in such a place, you can meditate anywhere, at anytime.

While I don't suggest you rush to the nearest noisy public place to meditate, I would like to tell you that you *can* meditate anywhere, not just at home. Try meditating on public transport, at the beach, in the bush, by a river, as a passenger on a boat, on an airplane, in hotels, resorts, retreats, on a rock, and pretty much anywhere you stop for a few minutes.

When I am driving, I often stop the car somewhere if it looks as though the sunset will be spectacular. I prefer a quiet spot with a good view and I either sit in the car, on the bonnet or on a bench, if there is one close by. I watch the sunset's kaleidoscope of shapes and colors. I imagine breathing in the sun's rays and the colors displayed so magnificently across the sky (see p.54–55 regarding breathing colours). It is a beautiful and peaceful thing to do, and it leaves me feeling refreshed and joyous.

What I do recommend when you meditate outside of your home is to use the white lighting exercise before you begin meditation. I think of it as a safe practice to protect you while you have your eyes closed. Naturally, if you are on public transport or in a public place, it makes sense to place your personal belongings in such a position that they can't be taken from you by unscrupulous characters. Other than this, you may find it useful to incorporate the noises around you into your meditation. Do not become irritated with the noises that other people make, but simply detach yourself from judgments and allow the noises to come in and out of your consciousness.

The main items you need for meditating are things such as a good straight-backed chair if sitting, a firm cushion for your head if lying down, a big cushion for the floor if sitting cross-legged, or a meditation stool. You may also need a shawl or jumper to keep you warm. Your body temperature will tend to drop a little when you meditate, so in cool weather, it's better to have something around your shoulders or wear something cozy so that the feeling of being chilled doesn't distract you from your meditation.

It is not necessary to rush out and buy anything special for meditation, you have all the things you need at home already. Remember the traditional image of an Indian yogi who dresses in a loincloth and doesn't mind where he meditates. The yogi has the simplest needs – somewhere to sleep and food to eat. He doesn't look for material things to bring happiness to his life. This is a difficult accomplishment in modern times, although some people do opt for the simpler life, believing it will alleviate feelings of dissatisfaction and restlessness. The message is, keep it simple. The main aim is to begin the practice of meditation without regarding the reasons you find as to why you are not ready. You are ready right now – it's simply a choice or decision, and once you begin you will wonder why on earth you didn't begin a long time ago.

Many people set aside a special area for their meditation, either a whole room or a quiet corner somewhere.

You can place the following items in your meditation space:

- a photograph or print which is meaningful to you;
- some scented or attractive candles;
- crystals (see p 56–63);
- an oil burner;
- little pieces of nature such as shells, stones, feathers, leaves or whatever you find on your travels;
- a beautiful cushion, shawl or rug;
- a box of essential oils (see p 64–71), candles and matches for your oil burner; or
- anything else that is meaningful to you and brings with it a sense of joy and peace.

Setting up a special place isn't a necessity, but if you can set up such a place and incorporate small rituals like the lighting of the candles and/or the oil burner, you will find yourself entering the meditative state more readily. A ritualistic way of beginning a meditation acts as a trigger for your mind to promote stillness.

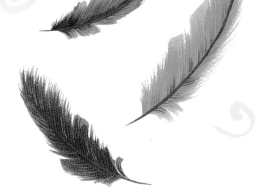

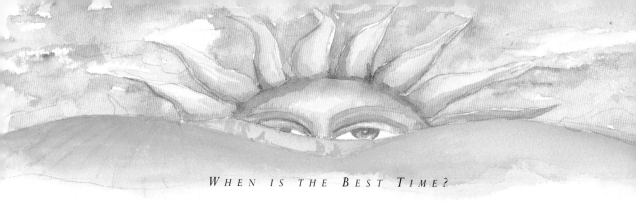

It is thought that the best time to meditate is early in the morning, around sunrise, or at sunset. It would be ideal if you could rise an hour or so earlier than you would usually and do some gentle exercise, such as walking, stretching or some simple relaxation exercises, which would be followed by a 20 minute (at least) meditation. For those who wake easily in the morning, this might be the best strategy.

If you are not a morning person, try doing your meditation at night. I like to meditate at night when I have done all I need to at home and can sit peacefully. If you meditate for extended periods late at night, say for an hour or more, you run the risk of feeling so revitalized that you may not be able to sleep well. However, if you meditate for up to 30 minutes, this should not present a problem, and you will actually sleep much more soundly.

Any time of day is suitable for meditating. Some of my friends prefer meditating during the day rather than at either end. This depends on your usual daily activities and where you can find the time and place.

Other people have such busy and stressful lives that they find the only time for meditating is on the bus or train, taking them to and from work. Whatever your situation, there are always a few minutes where a short meditation can be included in your schedule. Try to make it a priority somewhere in your day to meditate for at least five to 10 minutes, preferably more.

I once attended a lecture by Dr Deepak Chopra, author of many books, including *The Seven Spiritual Laws Of Success*. He said that you must practice something once a day for a month before it becomes a habit. If you meditate daily for a month, by the month's end, meditation will feel like an important part of your day.

Meditation practice – sunrise or sunset meditation

This meditation is ideal if you can sit facing the rising or setting sun, focussing on the changing light. If you only have time to meditate during the day, you may want to focus on the sky and the trees around you. You can also use the moon for your meditations at night – focussing on the moon and its rays.

First, do the relaxation and white lighting exercises. Allow your breathing to become soft and regular.

Second, if doing a meditation during sunrise or sunset, use the changing sunlight and its colors as your focus. Imagine that the light and colors are surrounding and soaking into your body. Feel the warmth of the sun's rays on your skin and watch the colors changing. If there are clouds in the sky, watch their shapes transform and drift past. Imagine that any worries or concerns you have melt with the sun's rays and dissipate into the air.

Close your eyes and breathe deeply, listening to all the sounds around you – the sounds that birds make at sunrise or sunset, the noise of insects and other sounds of life near you. See yourself connected with all living things and feel the peace this brings.

Allow all the muscles in your body to soften and relax and then open your eyes to see the sky once again. Imagine that the energy from the sun is regenerating your own energy, leaving you feeling refreshed and centered.

When you meditate at home, you are likely to encounter all manner of distractions – doorbells, the telephone, dogs barking, children crying, lawnmowers, cars starting, doors slamming, neighbors' music, airplanes flying overhead and any other number of regular occurrences in your neighborhood.

First and foremost, you must accept that these things will occur and may distract you. Do not allow yourself to become irritated by them because such feelings are totally unproductive. What you can do is make arrangements to manage the distractions that are within your control. Put on the answering machine for the telephone or ask those you live with to take messages for you. Hang a sign on the front door saying something like "stepped out for 10 minutes". This way visitors will not ring the doorbell and will hopefully return when you will be "home" again. If you live with others, ask them to answer the door and make apologies for your absence until you have finished your meditation.

It is a good idea to talk to those you live with about your need to meditate and the length of time you require for your meditation. Ask them not to disturb you unless it is absolutely crucial and ask for their support in your endeavors. If you have children you may need to explain to them why you cannot be disturbed and ask them to help you with your special time. If they are very young, you may need to ask a friend or neighbour to mind them for half an hour once a week. You can even teach them some of the techniques – you can never learn meditation too young.

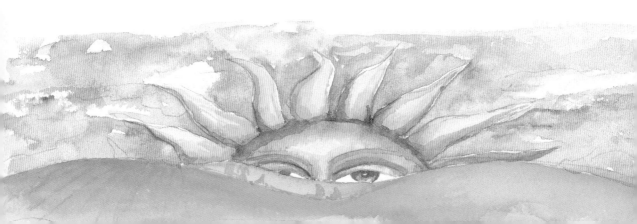

As for outside noises beyond your control, try incorporating them into your meditation as part of the focus. For example, if your neighbor starts a lawn-mower, focus on the sound of the lawnmower motor. Listen to the way it revs higher when being pushed over thick grass and how the revs drop when being pushed over short grass.

You can make a meditation out of any regular noise. I used to attend yoga classes years ago in a building on a very busy road. The teacher would have her students concentrate on the noise of the vehicles. We would pick one vehicle that was far up the road, listen to it coming closer and closer, then listen to it driving past and then further and further away until it could not be heard any longer. If you live near an airport, you can apply this technique for managing the sound of airplanes coming and going.

The same technique can be applied to barking dogs. Listen to the timbre and pitch of one dog's bark and then focus on another one (if there is more than one dog joining in). Allow the sounds of the barking to waft in and out of your consciousness and do not allow yourself to become judgmental of the noise.

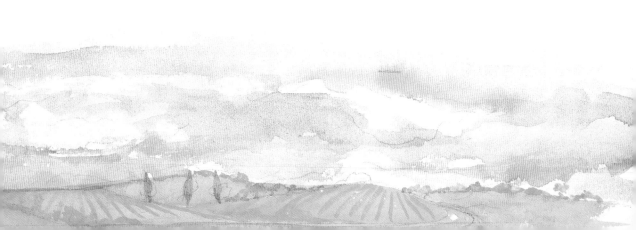

Meditative Techniques for Every Day

W e live incredibly busy lives, attending to all manner of needs for our jobs, family, friends, pets and homes, and it's not often that we allow time for ourselves. Soon the stress we feel mentally manifests itself into physical form within our bodies with the muscles usually the first to suffer. With the added stress of little or no exercise, or perhaps too much exercise, our muscles become stiff and sore. When this occurs we suffer from headaches, an aching back, aching limbs, digestive problems, a stiff neck, poor range of movement in our shoulders and arms, and general stiffness throughout our bodies.

The following exercise can be practiced anywhere and anytime, and takes just a few minutes. It's ideal to do at work several times a day and it helps you to bring yourself back to being really present and in the moment.

The breath is one of the most important relaxation tools we have. We generally breathe without paying much attention to how we breathe. A little stress leaves us breathing with shallow breaths and without exhaling all the air left in our lungs. Basically, we spend most of our time a little deprived of decent amounts of oxygen, and when we consciously breathe deeply we bring to our bodies and minds a sense of greater relaxation.

You will notice, when you try the exercise below, what effect simply stopping for a few minutes and bringing your attention to your body and breathing has on your state of mind. It is then apparent how our breaths are shallow and how our minds are cluttered. Do this exercise anytime to help you bring yourself back into the moment.

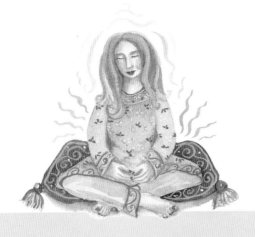

Body scan and breathing exercise

Sit with your feet flat on the floor and your hands in your lap. Close your eyes and spend a few seconds noticing how you are breathing. Is your breath shallow, deep, or is it rapid? Spend a few seconds doing a "body scan", noticing the areas of tension or discomfort in your body. How relaxed are your shoulders? Is your neck stiff? Does your stomach feel tense?

How are your stress and anxiety levels? Are you worrying about something you can do nothing about just at the moment? Are you feeling overwhelmed by the demands placed upon you?

Now spend a minute or two breathing in and out deeply and slowly, so that both your chest and abdomen fully expand and contract. When breathing out, be sure to exhale all the air from your lungs before breathing in again. Watch your breath fill the areas of discomfort in your body, surrounding, softening and releasing the tension. Adjust your posture and shoulders, and move your neck and arms to release the tightness.

Now spend a few seconds noticing how you feel mentally and physically. Are you more relaxed? Have your shoulders dropped a little and softened? If you don't feel any better at all, repeat the exercise once or twice more, making further improvements to your posture each time.

What kinds of mundane activities do you do during an average day? Here's a list of common things we may all do:

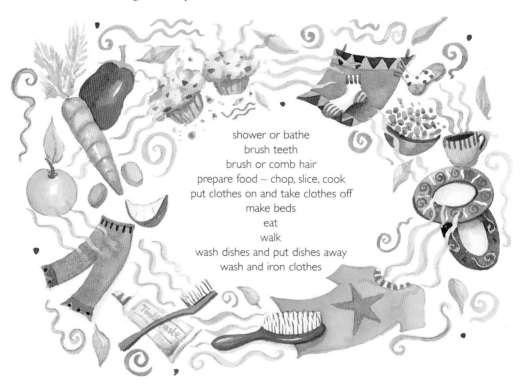

shower or bathe
brush teeth
brush or comb hair
prepare food – chop, slice, cook
put clothes on and take clothes off
make beds
eat
walk
wash dishes and put dishes away
wash and iron clothes

To live consciously does not mean that your awareness should only be enhanced during the time you meditate. In fact, to bring awareness into the mundane tasks you perform brings you back into the present moment time and again each day.

With each and every task you do, bring your attention to your breath and actions. For example, while brushing your teeth, think about what you are doing, notice how the bristles feel on your gums, how the toothpaste smells and tastes

Mindful dressing exercise

Do this exercise if you have just bathed and are about to dress. Take a few minutes to gather all the clothes you will be wearing. As you put on the first piece of clothing notice its texture, smell, color and how it feels against your skin. Notice the sensations as you pull the clothing on. Do this with each piece of clothing, being aware of every sensation and the reaction of your senses – touch, smell, feel and sound. It may take a minute or two longer to dress because you will naturally become a little slower in your actions so that you can savor the sensations.

You can use this technique for any activity – allowing all your senses to be heightened by being mindful.

and what sounds the toothbrush makes against your teeth. Bring all your attention to the actions you make and the reactions of your senses.

How often do you take notice of what you are doing when carrying out these tasks? How long has it been since you ate consciously? We are often so busy in our minds that we chew in accordance with how quickly our thoughts are whizzing through – FAST. It's no wonder so many people suffer with digestive disturbances. We need to take some time when we eat so that the food is thoroughly chewed and so that the digestive processes occur efficiently. Digestion begins in the mouth, so if the food spends too a short a time there, it is not processed enough before going onto the next phase in the stomach.

Many digestive problems can be reduced by mindful eating. For a start, mindful eating slows your thoughts and then brings with it some relaxation, which benefits your digestion.

Imagine if you were mindful when doing all kinds of activities during the day. A greater improvement in general well-being would occur because you would often be in a meditative state.

Every now and then we get caught in traffic jams or have to stand in queues for many long minutes waiting to be served. Sometimes the stress this causes is almost unbearable and we can literally feel the anxiety level rise. When we are already stressed, a delay such as this can lead us to having an angry outburst through sheer frustration.

Have you ever experienced this? Have you ever realised, after your angry or tearful outburst, just how emotionally uncentered or unbalanced you are? This is when you finally recognize that you need some relaxation or a break. However, if you were meditating or allowing yourself a few minutes' "time out" every day, you would be much less likely to reach such a state so readily.

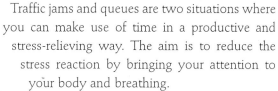

Traffic jams and queues are two situations where you can make use of time in a productive and stress-relieving way. The aim is to reduce the stress reaction by bringing your attention to your body and breathing.

When you find yourself feeling stressful over being in either of these situations, stop and ask yourself if there is anything feasible you can do to hurry the queue or sidestep the traffic. If there is something you can do, do it. If there is nothing you can do, you need to accept that this is one of those situations that you cannot change. Allow yourself the peace of letting go of your expectations. Don't sit or stand there with your breathing becoming more shallow and your heart rate speeding.

Follow the exercise opposite to release the tension from your mind and body, and simply

'Forget the jams and queues' exercise

Here you are in a traffic jam or standing in a queue. First, evaluate your breathing – is it shallow? Take three long, slow, deep breaths and do a body scan to sense where you are holding tension. While breathing deeply and rhythmically, systematically work through your muscles, tensing and relaxing each muscle group.

Start with your shoulders, moving them forwards and backwards until you feel the muscles loosen. Tighten all the muscles in your arms and make hard fists with your hands. Hold for a few seconds and then release. Clench your buttock muscles and tighten your tummy muscles for several seconds and then release. Tighten all the muscles in your legs from top to bottom for a few seconds and then release. Gently rotate each foot, pointing your toes and then flexing your foot to loosen the muscles in your feet. Now take several more deep breaths and evaluate your body once again.

If you are still in the jam or queue, repeat the exercise or just concentrate on your breathing.

let yourself be in the present moment without worrying about what else you could be doing. While simplistic, you can apply these principles to any situation over which you just don't have any control. Once you have evaluated what you can do to improve the situation and then surrendered yourself to an acceptance of what you cannot change, your mind will relax. Once your mind relaxes, your body will follow.

How many times have you had so much to do that you felt as though you could not function properly because you were anxious about achieving all your goals? You didn't know where to start, which task had priority and, when you did begin, your mind couldn't concentrate and your thoughts tumbled around chaotically.

To stop the chaos, you need to recognise the symptoms. These can be as mild as feeling a little stressed and anxious or as urgent as feeling on the verge of an emotional breakdown. Shallow breathing, increased heart rate, fast palpitations, sweating, tummy upset, headache, tense shoulders, stiff neck, panic attacks, confusion, depression, feeling that you are on the verge of tears, angry outbursts and feeling violent are all symptoms of "dis-stress".

If you relate to this category, you need to take action. Evaluate your situation and decide if you can take a few minutes to go for a walk around the block. Immediate improvements can be made by taking just a few minutes to do a short meditation or, at least, some deep breathing.

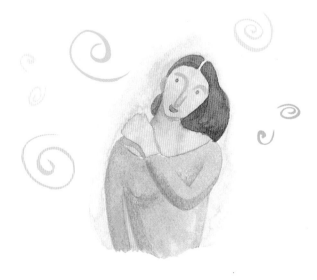

Your comment will be, "Well if I am over-stressed, then how will I fit in a meditation?" A logical question, but you are not achieving anything by not looking after yourself. Three to five minutes is the least you can give yourself.

Follow the very simple exercise below whenever you feel chaotic, or better still, use it to prevent ever feeling too chaotic. In my classes, I suggest that my students practice this exercise daily sometime during the course of their working day. The exercise helps you become centered or maintain a feeling of being centered when heavy demands are being placed upon you.

'Stop the chaos' exercise

STOP. Wherever you are, at work or at home – STOP STILL. Focus on your breathing and evaluate it. Is your breathing shallow?

Concentrate on breathing slowly and deeply. Close your eyes and imagine yourself in one of your favorite outdoor places – by the sea, in a rain forest, in a park, by a river, in the wilderness, on a boat, or wherever. The place is somewhere you have been before and where you have experienced a sense of peace, relaxation or joy.

Imagine yourself in this place and bring to mind every little detail. The sights, sounds, smells, fragrances, touch, and – if applicable – tastes. Then recall the feeling of peace you experienced there in minute detail. Imagine feeling that way right now. Relive the feelings and feel that energy flow into your body and mind. Relive the sense of being carefree and relaxed. Watch your breathing and focus on breathing deeply and slowly, allowing the breath to travel freely around your body.

Now go back to your tasks with this feeling of relaxation and with a lighter perspective.

One skill we tend to lose touch with when overly stressed or unbalanced is the skill of being objective with our dealings with others. I feel this is essential for reducing conflict and maintaining a feeling of being centered.

Let us look at objectivity a little more closely. What is objectivity? It is the ability to relate to others without becoming affected by personal bias or emotions. This may sound as if I am suggesting you be cold and indifferent to others but that is not the case. To be objective is to be able to step "out of the picture" and be more detached emotionally so that you can "respond" to the other person rather than "react".

We all have buttons that, when pressed by the comments or demands of others, elicit in us what is called a "knee-jerk reaction". This is usually an uncomfortable reaction that brings with it feelings of inferiority, inadequacy, anger, fear or anxiety. All of these feelings throw us off-center and disturb our ability to feel peaceful. Fear is usually at the bottom of these reactions: fear of rejection, ridicule, being taken for granted, being used, losing face, being inadequate, losing love, being unloved, and giving too much. They are all seemingly valid fears, but the creation of inharmonious relations because of fear will only exacerbate the fears and their harmful effect.

To achieve objectivity you need to maintain a centered state so that you can become more of an observer in these situations. To observe involves looking at all the people involved in the interaction with detachment. For example, if you always argue with your partner or a close relative, step onto the observer's platform and look at yourself and them without judgment, and with compassion and empathy. Step into the other person's shoes to see what fears or emotions cause them to act in such a fashion. And then look at yourself, considering the underlying causes of your reactions.

Communicating with compassion helps you to relate in a more loving way. It reduces your uncomfortable reactions considerably and brings to your relationships a deeper bond and closeness. This applies to any dealings you have with others. We have all had to cope with the inappropriate behavior of others in work

Objectivity exercise

Sit quietly and, for several minutes, focus on breathing deeply and slowly. Think of a time when you were relating with someone in a way that caused emotional discomfort. Replay the "movie" of this interaction in detail, reliving all the emotions you experienced at the time.

Imagine yourself stepping onto the "observer's platform", and watch the movie again without judgment and with compassion for both the people on the screen. Look closely at the person who is interacting with you and consider where their fears lie, why they were speaking to you in that fashion and why they reacted the way they did. Then look closely at your role – what were your fears, what made you react in the way you did?

Replay the entire scene, replacing your dialogue and behavior with that of compassion and love coming from a state of objectivity and detachment. See how the other person would then respond, rather than react, to your considered words and how you would inevitably have a more harmonious interaction.

or social situations. When I see people behaving aggressively, my first thought is to wonder what they are fearful of, or what is going on in their life which makes them act in such a way. I try not to allow my ego to jump in to make me feel indignant, or cause a reaction without thought. To first consider your response in these situations in such a way is a liberating experience. It frees you from having to be involved emotionally and allowing the situation to drain your energy. It gives you the space to consider how you would like to respond, and to decide whether you really need to respond at all.

To help you develop this skill in your life, use the exercise above on a regular basis. Use the many scenarios you have already experienced to practice objectivity. If you become involved in an upsetting conversation with someone, use this exercise to see how it could have been avoided and then use the skills next time you need them – during the actual conversation.

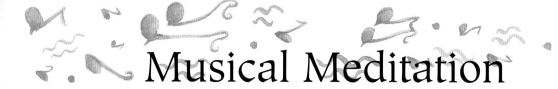

Musical Meditation

The ability of music to soothe or enchant the soul is well known. Without music we would probably not experience as much joy and happiness in our lives. Consider for a moment a world without music – what would replace the music we love to hear? Would opera merely be performers speaking poetically on stage? What would build the anticipation in a horror movie if there was no dramatic music accompanying the scenes? How would singers convey their sentiments of love and tragedy without music to match their mood? In what way would we express happiness and well-being if we couldn't whistle or hum a favorite tune while going about our daily tasks?

Music brings with it so many emotions – the full gamut of human experience can be related to it. How many times have you heard a song or piece of music and a memory has been brought to mind? The music acts as a trigger for your memories and emotions. Think of an important event in your life and consider what music or song reminds you of that time. I can think of countless experiences where a particular piece of music has transported me back in time.

Now think of the music you most like to listen to and consider which type of music or which artist triggers feelings of well-being and harmony in your mind and body. It is well worth taking a look at the compact discs, tapes and/or records you own to piece together a range of music which makes you feel happy and content. Play this music often to encourage this state of mind, particularly when you need a lift, or when you feel overwhelmed.

The style of music that makes you feel good is very personal and may not appeal to other people in the same way. Just become familiar with your own special music and try not to allow the possible disapproval of others to lessen your enjoyment. You may have to use headphones or a Walkman if those you live with don't gain the same pleasure from your music.

Use the music awareness exercise on page 45 to gain a greater appreciation of your music and to listen with more awareness.

Some types of music are not likely to impart feelings of harmony. In fact, some types of music can be jarring and can raise your blood pressure, or increase feelings of agitation. If you are feeling stressed, you may feel more sensitive to this type of music. I recall times when I have been shopping and have had to leave the store because the music played there made me feel agitated. While shop owners can't possibly hope to please everyone with their musical selections, there are certain types of music that do irritate many people. On the other hand there are certain types of music that can create a feeling of well-being.

Shopping malls tend to bombard us with noise on many levels. Apart from the music each store may play, there is the music played in the general part of the mall as well as the announcements made by various promoters advertising their latest specials and deals. On top of that, we are exposed to the "life noises" of the shoppers, such as children screaming or crying and people talking loudly. Underlying this cacophony are the sounds of air-conditioning units, escalators and lifts. Have you ever felt totally drained after a shopping expedition? Now you know why – all this noise can create havoc in your mind and can increase your stress levels profoundly. I have a friend who listens to calming music on his Walkman while he goes shopping to drown out all the noise he finds intolerable.

The type of music that promotes a feeling of harmony is melodic and flowing. It doesn't matter whether you choose classical, new age or music by your favourite instrumentalist, providing the music gives you a feeling of tranquility. It is best not to use music with words as they may trigger thoughts or memories. The exception is when the words are sung in a language that you don't understand, making the words become merely a collection of sounds. Opera music could be enjoyed in this way.

Don't listen to music that is discordant unless you find it particularly soothing. Melodic classical and new age music are good choices. If you feel especially deprived of nature, music incorporating natural sounds can be calming.

Look in the classical and new age sections of your music store and ask to listen to some of the music you find appealing – before making your selection.

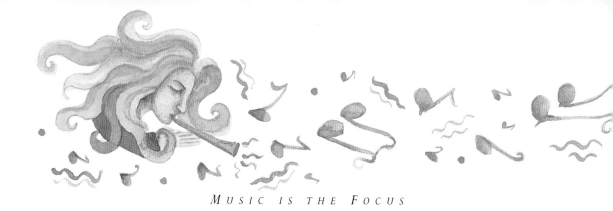

MUSIC IS THE FOCUS

Music can be used in meditation as your focus. Play the music and choose any meditation position that is comfortable and which you will not fall asleep in. Concentrate on every sound and every pause between the notes. Some people may find the music is distracting during their meditation while others find it perfect for stilling a busy mind. Experiment with different types of music before you come to any conclusions on how you enjoy this style of meditation.

Music such as Gregorian chants and others found in different yogic philosophies may appeal to you. Siddha yoga ashrams often have a store where you can buy tapes of their traditional chants. Call your closest ashram for details. Alternatively, a search on the Internet may also uncover some interesting web sites.

The exercise opposite outlines how to use music during your meditation to help you focus your mind.

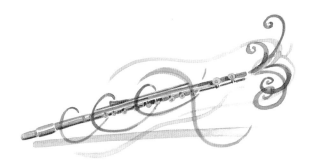

Music awareness exercise

After doing the relaxation and white lighting exercises (see pp 19 and 21) put on your favorite compact disc, tape or record and sit or lie quietly listening to the music. Imagine that you are in front of the band or orchestra and picture every person playing their instrument. Concentrate on one of the instruments being played and hear the notes it plays. Picture the person playing this one instrument. What does the instrument look like? What pitch does it play?

Then move on to the next instrument and picture it being played, noticing the play of notes within the music. Focus on the rest of the instruments being played, one by one.

Focus on any other sounds in the music — the sound of a person singing or of the nature sounds — and notice the nuances of each sound.

If your mind begins to wander, imagine the distracting thoughts drifting away on clouds into the sky and gently bring your mind back to the music.

Finish the exercise with several deep and slow breaths bringing yourself back to the room by wiggling your fingers and toes. Open your eyes and sit quietly for a few minutes, revelling in the stillness in your mind.

Colorful Meditation

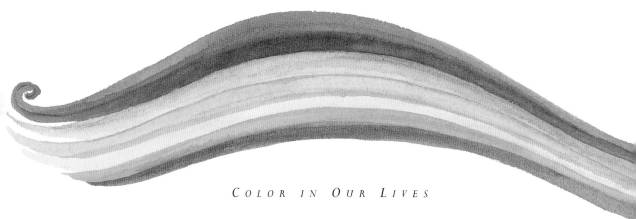

Our lives would be deadly dull and boring without color giving us a sense of zest and vibrancy. Imagine a world where everything was gray, including the fruit, vegetables, trees, plants and everything else we eat and use. Sounds dreadful, doesn't it? Can you picture a sunrise or sunset of different gray tones, or perhaps a beach scene where all things are various shades of gray? We take color for granted but without it we would surely shrivel.

Some of the poorest regions in the world seem bright and lively because their peoples choose to dress in brilliant colors, almost as if they are making up for their poverty by bringing color into their lives. India, Tibet, Peru, Africa and Thailand come to mind — their national dress is made of the brightest and most eye-catching colored fabrics.

Color plays such an important role in creating the various moods and emotions we experience. We even use color in our general conversation. "I was green with envy", "I saw red – I was so angry", "I just feel a bit blue today", and "I'm in black mood", are just a few commonly used references linking color to emotion.

You may not be aware of the fact that product manufacturers have marketing teams who make decisions on the best colors for product packaging and point of

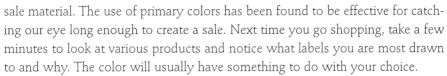

sale material. The use of primary colors has been found to be effective for catching our eye long enough to create a sale. Next time you go shopping, take a few minutes to look at various products and notice what labels you are most drawn to and why. The color will usually have something to do with your choice.

Think of color as energy and then think of each color containing a different type of energy which can affect our emotions and our state of mind in various ways. For example, you may wake one morning and feel a bit flat but you know you will have a busy day at the office. To give yourself a lift, you may wear a color such as red, orange or hot pink. These colors not only make you look vibrant, but add a certain energy to your state of mind, helping you get through the day's activities with a positive force. This is not your imagination, it is the energy that the color promotes.

Your colors exercise

Spend some time looking at your home and jot down the main colors you have used for your decor. What color are your favorite clothes? Looking at all your belongings, what color are the items that make you feel peaceful? Hold various colors up against your skin and look in the mirror to evaluate which ones bring out your coloring and features the best. Take note of any color that you simply do not like.

Color has been shown to affect the growth rate of plants. A study was carried out on the effects of colored light when growing mustard cress from seeds. The cress grown under a pure red light had stunted growth and was not healthy, and the cress grown under a pure green light was weak and poor growing. However, the cress grown under a pure blue light was well developed, slow growing and tasted sweet.

It has been shown that each color emits an energy vibration that can be picked up regardless of sight abilities. In fact, blind people can, with practice, pick various colors by learning the differing vibrations and "feeling" them by touch. This demonstrates the possibilities associated with using color in therapy and how color therapy can be grouped with vibrational medicine.

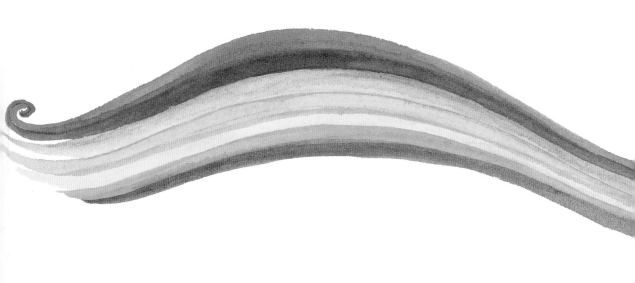

Getting in touch with color exercise

Sit quietly and do the relaxation and white lighting exercises. Concentrate on your breathing, making your breaths deep and slow. While you are breathing, imagine that the air you are breathing is colored – choose the first color that comes to mind. Just sit quietly and meditate on your breath and the color. Notice if you see the color on your "mind screen" and also if the color you breathe changes. Do this for several minutes and then turn to *What the colors mean* to evaluate where you may need rebalancing. Our minds tend to choose the colors we need to help rebalance our energies.

Color is used in therapy as a means of gaining an understanding of a person's emotional well-being. The human aura is made up of layers of different colored energy which surround the entire body. Therapists who read auras take note of areas of discoloration and leakage of energy. They then use various means to rebalance their client's energy, such as crystals, silk fabrics, meditation, color visualization and essential oils made from colorful plants. Color used in this fashion helps to bring about new feelings and stimulates different emotions and thoughts, creating a sense of inner harmony.

Art therapists encourage their clients to use color as a means of expression. The client reveals their emotions through the artwork they produce. The therapist then helps the person to verbalize the issues that have manifested through their creativity. It is a non-confrontational form of therapy which enlists the support of the creative mind to highlight important emotional struggles.

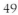

Red is the color of power and action. It is a warming color and represents vitality, sexuality and high energy. Red spurs us into action by increasing our motivation and aggression – think of the saying "it was like waving a red rag to a bull". It is an excellent color to use when your energy levels are low and fatigue has set in. However, too much of a good thing can turn into a destructive force by becoming overly aggressive, too emotional, pushy or too sexually charged. As this color is thought to increase blood pressure, it should probably be avoided by those with heart problems – don't go mad with red decor in this case. Red in an office setting is not very conducive to harmonious relationships and could trigger off a feeling of anger in stressed employees.

Blue, on the other hand, is calming and encourages feelings of peace. It is the color of serenity and protection and promotes restful sleep. The image of a peaceful blue ocean beneath a serene blue sky dotted with fluffy white clouds is one that easily prompts a feeling of calmness. As blue is a cool color, it is best 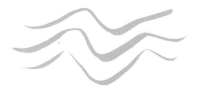 not used in great quantities by people who feel the cold easily. However, it is excellent for those people who feel the heat. Too much blue, especially deeper blues, can bring out feelings of insecurity and fear in particularly sensitive people. Blue also encourages a sense of quiet and contemplation, so it is an excellent color to have in and around your meditation corner.

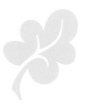 **Green** is a predominant color in nature and there are many shades represented in the plants and trees of the world. It is full of healing and harmonious vibrations and is a balancing color that will help restore self-esteem and hope after emotional upsets. Green is often used in healing color meditations for diseases, such as cancer, and it works alongside blue to restore health to the body.

Too much green may create so much tranquility that a person's natural drive and motivation is reduced. To counteract this, add a few touches of bright color to balance the energies.

Yellow, the color of consciousness, brings with it happy and joyous thoughts. Imagine a field of sunflowers and you will understand the thoughts this sunny color provokes. In my classes, I show different pictures of flowers and nature which represent the various colors. The picture of a sun-flower always provokes a smile or two in the class and I can  sense a change in my students' energy levels. Use this warm color to uplift, increase concentration, promote liveliness and boost communication. Always use a bright, pure yellow in meditation and in your decor. Too much yellow may create excessive chatter in talkative people, but combined with blue or green this tendency can be balanced.

 **Brown** occurs in many shades, from the color of a peanut shell to the richness of chestnut brown, and is a strong and earthy color which is excellent for grounding flighty people. It is represented throughout nature and, if drawn to this color, you may feel the need to have your feet on the earth. Too much brown can bring one's ener-gy too far down into the earth and make one insensitive to the emotional aspects of life. As with all things, bal-ance is the key, and it is wise to blend browns with light, uplifting colors such as yellow, green and orange.

Pink is the color of love and healing. It is a combination of red and white, and subdues and balances qualities of both these colors. The darker and brighter the pink, the more energetic and aggressive it becomes, while the softer pinks reflect more the softness of white.

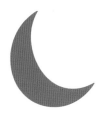

Violet is a color of dignity and beauty which increases feelings of self-respect and self-esteem. This beautiful color is linked with spirituality and creativity. Its energy is quite strong and may be too strong for some people who are not open to its force. For this reason, use it with a soft green to balance this energy.

Magenta represents spiritual energy and is excellent for helping you step away from obsessive behaviour and thoughts. Being a strong color, its energy is quite dramatic, bringing with it a sensuous quality and a sense of motivation. Use this color when you need to develop emotional independence, or when you need to let go of certain reminiscences or obsessive thoughts.

Orange is a color that uplifts and brings joy and fun. It brings greater courage and helps you make life-changing decisions and actions. For this reason it resolves feelings of restlessness and the lack of direction or vitality. However, too much orange can actually increase feelings of restlessness by making a person seek change too often. Balance with green.

Turquoise, being a mix of green and blue, provides a beautiful blend of two special colors. It is useful for boosting immune function and reducing inflammation. The atmosphere it creates is one of peace and tranquility, and it promotes a carefree outlook.

Indigo is a color connected to higher energies and, with positive use, it increases spirituality and intuition. Indigo also helps increase self-confidence and self-esteem. Being a deep blue, it has a strong energy, so if you are often drawn to wearing and using this color, balance it with soft pink or lemon.

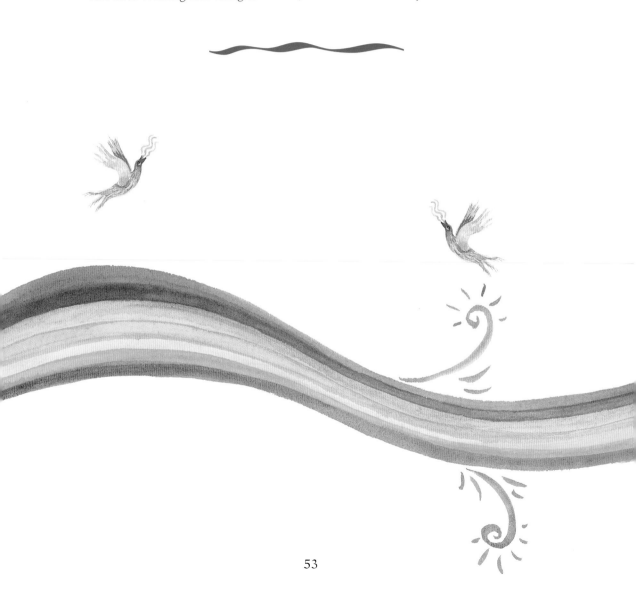

Colored ball meditation

There are many ways to use color in meditation and all methods are successful in bringing changes in mood and temperament. These are the various methods:

• The breathing color form of meditation (see p 49).

• The object focus technique (see p. 15) and choose an object which is colored in a way that appeals to you. Imagine yourself being surrounded by and "steeped" in the color of the object as you focus upon it.

• Imagine sitting in a ball of the color you most need and see that color soaking into your body and filling every cell (much like the white lighting exercise on p 21).

• Tape and follow the colored ball meditation outlined opposite.

First do the relaxation and white lighting exercises and then sit quietly for a few minutes while focussing on your breath.

Imagine a ball of brilliant red energy spinning by the side of your left foot. Watch the ball slowly spin and move upwards along the left side of your body. See it pass along your lower leg, thigh and left buttock, and then watch it travel up the side of your body, alongside your arm, neck and head and then see it travel in through the top of your head and then down the center of your body to finish at the base of your spine, where you leave it softly spinning in the one spot.

Now, imagine a ball of brilliant orange energy spinning by the side of your right foot. Watch the ball slowly spin and move upwards along the right side of your body. See it pass along your lower leg, thigh and right buttock, and then watch it travel up the side of your body, alongside your arm, shoulder, neck and head and then see it travel in through the top of your head and then down the center of your body to finish at the place just behind your navel, where you leave it softly spinning in the one spot.

Then imagine a ball of brilliant yellow-gold energy spinning in front of your feet. See it travel slowly, spinning, upwards along the front of your body, following each and every contour. See it enter the crown of your head and travel down through your body until it reaches your solar plexus, where you leave it softly spinning in the one spot.

See a ball of brilliant green energy spinning at the back of your feet. Watch it travel slowly, spinning upwards, along the back of your body, following all the contours. See it enter the crown of your head and travel down through your body until it reaches the center of your chest, where you leave it softly spinning in the one spot.

Watch a ball of brilliant blue energy spinning at the top of your head and then see it slowly wind clockwise downwards around your body while softly spinning. See it travelling down past your head, neck, shoulders, arms, torso, buttocks, thighs, lower legs and towards the bottom of your feet. Watch the brilliant blue color enter the base of your feet to travel upwards through your legs and then through your body to finish in your throat area, where you leave it softly spinning in the one spot.

See a ball of brilliant indigo energy spinning at the base of your feet and watch it slowly wind clockwise upwards around your body while softly spinning. See it travel up past your lower legs, thighs, buttocks, torso, arms, shoulders, neck and to the top of your head. Then watch it enter the crown of your head to stop just behind the center of your forehead, where you leave it softly spinning in the one spot.

Imagine a ball of brilliant violet energy spinning softly beneath your feet and then see it enter the bottom of your feet, soaking into each and every cell as it travels softly through your body, filling and expanding as it travels upwards. See the violet energy soaking through your entire body and then gathering together in a ball of brilliant spinning energy at the top of your head.

See all the balls of color spinning softly, the red at the base of your spine, the orange behind your navel, the yellow-gold in your solar plexus, the green in the center of your chest, the blue in your throat area, the indigo behind the center of your forehead and the violet at the top of your head. Watch all the balls of energy increase in vibrancy and then watch them expand wider and wider until your body is surrounded by softly spinning colors.

Sit quietly for a few minutes in this powerful energy, allowing the colors to rebalance and revitalize every part of your body, mind and spirit.

Crystals in Meditation

HOW CRYSTALS WORK

To understand the energy in crystals we must remember how much energy and time has gone into their creation. Because they have a crystalline structure, they are able to collect and emit electromagnetic energy.

In ancient times, crystals were considered invaluable for use in healing, prayer and to increase spiritual connection. Admired for their beauty, crystals have been crafted into jewellery and used as decoration for thousands of years.

In one study conducted in the United States in the 1970s, over two hundred people suffering with pain held a crystal in their hand and the majority reported an almost immediate reduction in their pain levels.

There are many different types of crystals in the world and each variety has specific qualities available for use in meditation. Generally, their color is a guide to how they may be of use. Natural crystals, made over millions of years, have much greater benefits than man-made crystals, so always choose natural crystals for your personal use.

Our bodies are surrounded by an electromagnetic field or aura which is influenced by other electromagnetic forces around us. Crystals harness the highest

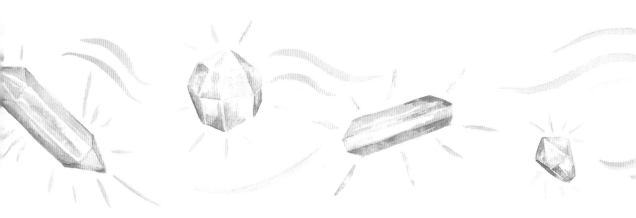

form of energy within their structure and emit this energy to those who wear them or who are close by. In this way they reharmonize imbalances in our aura, bringing us a greater sense of well-being.

When choosing crystals, use your intuition. Look at all the crystals on offer and choose the one or ones that you feel most drawn to. Do not analyze the reasons you feel more drawn to a particular crystal; trust your innate wisdom. You can also hold your hand over all the crystals and choose the one that promotes the strongest tingling feeling in the palm of your hand.

Realize too that on different days you may feel drawn to different crystals, depending on what you are experiencing in your life at the time and what energy you need to work with. Purchase several crystals to use at home or the workplace and re-evaluate your choices from time to time as your needs change.

You may like to keep some crystals within your home to create specific energy in various rooms. Study the list in *The basic crystals for meditation,* which outlines the crystals most beneficial for this work.

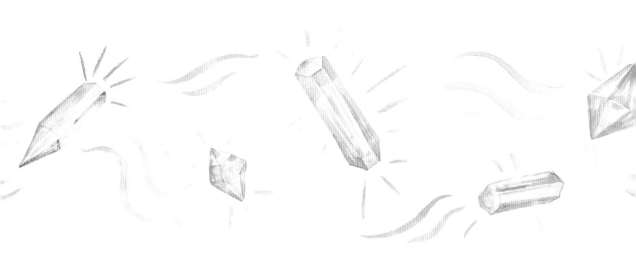

Agates are members of the chalcedony family of crystals. They are found in various colors and are translucent. The blue variety is calming, moss agate has especially grounding qualities, and red agate helps to energize the body. Across the board, agates are stabilizing, balancing, and work to increase self-acceptance and consciousness.

Amethyst is violet to purple in color and is a wonderful quartz crystal to meditate with as it is calming and increases powers of intuition. It is often used in healing and helps to correct problems with insomnia when kept under or near the pillow. Amethyst increases clarity of mind and is useful when changing negative thought patterns.

Aquamarine is a blue-green colored stone also known as the "water stone". This crystal also reduces negativity, promotes a feeling of courage, increases creativity, strengthens perception and intuition, and allows for greater inner calm and tranquility. It has the ability to strengthen the body's organs responsible for cleansing and purification.

Carnelian, like agate, is part of the chalcedony family and is a type of quartz available in abundance. Its colors range from red to orange and can sometimes exhibit a dark brown hue. It has grounding qualities which can help you tune into the Earth's energy. Carnelian has stimulating qualities which increase positive motivation while also easing stress and anxiety. Used in meditation, it brings greater happiness and helps you realize your dreams by encouraging you to follow your life's true path.

Diamonds are not only "a girl's best friend", but they also hold strong energy to help you increase spiritual awareness, willpower and courage. When used in meditation, they steer you away from a materialistic focus to the realization of higher truths as they connect you to the universal energy. When used in conjunction with other crystals, the diamond will strengthen the other crystals' qualities.

Emeralds are from the beryl family of stones and can be found in colors ranging from pale to very deep green. For meditation use, it is thought the paler emeralds hold the highest energy. The emerald is believed to be the stone of true love, increasing one's capacity for giving and receiving love and helps those who work in the healing professions to maintain emotional balance. This stone also improves self-esteem and memory, increases inspiration and intuition, is excellent for spiritual growth, and is soothing and calming.

Lapis lazuli is a deep blue stone which was used in ancient Egypt for decoration and spiritual rituals. It is has energizing qualities and helps to improve communication, creativity and mental focus. Used in meditation it helps one attain spiritual enlightenment and the understanding of universal truths. If wearing this stone, always place it above your diaphragm so that your energy is drawn upwards. Ideally, wear this stone around or near your throat area.

Moonstones are milky, translucent stones with flashes of pale blue or green. Another balancing crystal, the moonstone helps to increase intuition and logic, and acts to balance emotions. Where a person is oversensitive or overly driven by desires, moonstone acts as a balancing agent.

Quartz crystals encompass a large group of stones made mostly of silicon dioxide. Clear quartz is ideal for healing work as it allows pure white light to pass through it unaltered. All types of quartz crystals contain a beautiful energy for increasing emotional peace and wisdom. They increase positivity and help you reach your highest potential.

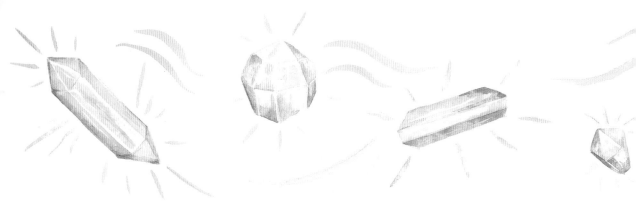

Rose quartz is a crystal infused with a soft pink color. It contains a gentle energy which promotes love and compassion. It has nurturing, feminine qualities which bring a sense of calm and awaken one's imagination. This crystal is beneficial at times of grieving and loss.

Sapphires are mostly deep blue in color but can also be found in gray, black, yellow or green. This mystical stone helps you to become at peace with the world and your life. It increases spiritual faith, good fortune and creativity, and helps you to concentrate.

Smoky quartz, as the name suggests, is a translucent crystal of a smoky brown color. This crystal helps to improve your temper, and alleviates mild depression and anxiety by encouraging the mind to think of new possibilities. It has positive and reassuring qualities and helps you become more in tune with environmental issues because of its connection with the Earth.

Tiger's eye is a glossy brown stone with golden stripes. It enhances self-confidence and helps us use our inner resources. It helps you unite your will and desire, bringing your ideas into reality. It is thought that tiger's eye brings to its wearer material possessions and helpful people.

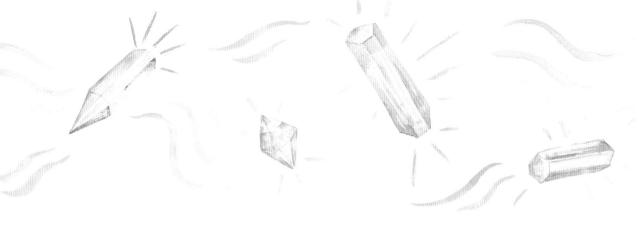

Topaz is a golden yellow or brown stone which is sometimes found in green or blue colors. This stone, like the sun, sends out healing rays of energy. It is a stone that brings inspiration and increases intuition and wisdom. It promotes tolerance and peace and helps you communicate more harmoniously with difficult people.

Tourmaline stones are a large group of stones which include black, blue, green, red, opalized, watermelon and cat's eye tourmaline. This group of stones encourages new perspectives and boosts confidence. A balancing quality enables this stone to help us find peace in our existence and to have useful insights. It brings calmness and clarity by dispelling negativity.

Turquoise is a beautiful stone that ranges from sky blue through bright blue to green blue. It has been used for jewellery since ancient times and is thought to help a person connect with their higher self. Turquoise possesses healing properties and can be used after surgery or to combat disease. It enhances friendship, communication and loyalty.

Meditating with crystals can be as simple as holding the crystal you are most drawn to in your hand while focussing on your breathing. Or it can be as elaborate as arranging a circle of crystals around your meditation place and then holding particular crystals for their specific qualities. A healing meditation can involve holding the crystal over the area of your body that is in need and then focussing on the crystal's energy pouring into your body to heal the tissues underneath.

You can use a crystal for its properties when you feel that you need balancing in a particular area of your life. In this way crystals help to release energy blocks which may be preventing you from moving forward.

If you feel your home or workplace contains negative energy, or if you have trouble settling down in these areas, you can use crystals to increase the positive energy and harmony surrounding you.

Try the meditation opposite and use the full power of your creative imagination to really "live" the words.

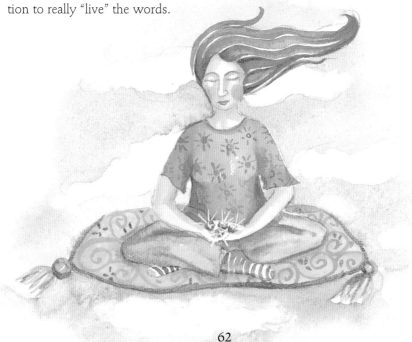

Crystal cave meditation

First do the relaxation and white lighting exercises (see page 21) and then sit quietly, focusing on breathing softly and deeply for several minutes.

See yourself walking along the bottom of a cliff face, with the magnificent ancient rock towering above you exuding the strength of the ages. As you walk along, you find the entrance to a cave and there is a soft, beautiful glow coming from within. Step inside and find yourself within a small cave high enough to stand upright in. Notice that there is a tunnel leading from the cave. As you walk through the tunnel, the mystical glow becomes brighter and you realize it is made of all the colors of the rainbow, swirling and intertwining around you. The air smells sweet, like the fragrance of flowers, and it is cool and refreshing.

As you come to the end of the tunnel you find yourself walking into another cave which is large and has walls covered with sparkling, brilliant crystals. The light emanating from the crystals is warm and comforting. You feel a palpable energy pouring around you, caressing your skin and hair with soft waves of light.

You notice a chair, decorated with many crystals, in the center of the cave. Sit in the chair and as you do so feel as if you have been enveloped in pure love and tranquility. Sit quietly, allowing the sensations to embrace your mind and heart. See the energy pouring into your body and soul.

Ask to be shown which crystal you need to increase your well-being and to address any issues you need assistance resolving or working through. The appropriate crystal will appear at your feet. Pick up the crystal and hold it in both hands in your lap, meditating on its powers. See the crystal energy dissolve your fears and help you move on to a better way of relating to yourself and others.

Now take the crystal with you, giving thanks, and leave the cave after memorizing all its details so that you can return at any time when you need guidance and peace.

Fragrant Meditation

ESSENTIAL OILS IN
MEDITATION

Pure essential oils derived from flowers, fruit, seeds, leaves, bark, roots and resin of plants and trees have been used since ancient times in spiritual and religious rituals, as perfume and for anointing. About 3,000 years ago, essential oils played a large role in Egypt, India and China. At the very least, these oils have the capacity to improve our feelings of well-being, and at the most, they play a part in healing body tissues. The tiny molecules of oil become absorbed into our bloodstream and work on psychological and physiological levels to improve our state of health.

Because the oils are so potent, they should never be applied directly to the skin, and great care must be taken with the quantities used. They are exquisite, and should not be used in a frivolous manner or without following directions. Do not think that if two drops of an oil is recommended that four or six would be even better. Essential oil blends are developed with specific safe quantities thoroughly considered.

As I shall be mainly discussing the use of oils with an oil burner, I urge you to find out the other physical applications of the oils for yourself through further investigation and reading.

Essential oils provide tremendous benefits when used in any medium, such as water or almond oil. If you are pregnant or suffer from epilepsy, you need to take special care in learning which oils you should avoid.

The list of oils in *The calming basics* include those which are ideal for meditation purposes. There are many more oils available and each oil has specific physical and psychological benefits. Look through the list and you may find that you are drawn to a particular oil which may be of use to you now.

The list below includes a number of oils particularly useful in meditation exercises and explains their psychological value as well as categorizing the scents as top, middle or base notes. The blending of these notes is discussed in *Blends*.

Basil *(Ocimum basilicum)* is helpful when you need to concentrate on a particular task. It helps us choose the best path or make the best decisions as we travel through life. Basil also eases depression, insomnia and anxiety. Do not use in pregnancy. TOP NOTE

Bergamot *(Citrus aurantium bergamia)* is a grounding oil which brings you into the present. It eases depression, stress, balances the emotions and calms the nerves. Bergamot has a high vibration and lifts the spirits, bringing a sense of increased happiness. TOP NOTE

Cedarwood *(Juniperus virginiana)* is used in an oil burner before and during meditation to help increase spiritual awareness. It soothes, eases depression and remedies insomnia. Do not use in pregnancy. BASE NOTE

Chamomile *(Anthemis nobilis, Matricaria chamomilla)* promotes calmness and relaxation and is excellent for meditation. It relieves stress, tension and depression, and helps to decrease insomnia. MIDDLE NOTE

Cinnamon *(Cinnamomum zeylanicum)* is a sweet-scented oil that increases spirituality and assists in the development of psychic abilities. It is thought that cinnamon increases abundance in our lives. MIDDLE NOTE

Fennel *(Foeniculum vulgare)* is an aniseed-scented oil that helps us find courage to make beneficial changes in our lives. It increases self-esteem and confidence. Do not use in pregnancy or if suffering from epilepsy. MIDDLE NOTE

Frankincense *(Boswellia thurifera)* is a most powerful oil to increase meditative experiences as it helps us to connect with the universal energy. This oil helps bring us into the present. BASE NOTE

Geranium *(Pelargonium graveolens)* is useful for protecting against and dispelling negative energy. It uplifts, relaxes and calms, and brings harmony and grace into our lives. MIDDLE NOTE

Jasmine *(Jasminum officinale)* uplifts and transforms your state of mind. It is a stimulant which acts as an aphrodisiac and relieves emotional suffering. It increases all types of love and is often used as a protecting agent. Jasmine is an excellent oil for easing a sense of pessimism and dispelling paranoia. BASE NOTE

Lavender *(Lavandula angustifolia, L. officinalis)* calms and harmonizes, balances the body and mind, and is useful in visualization to help strengthen all aspects of the self. This is a good oil to use if you suffer from mood swings and irritability. MIDDLE NOTE

Lemon *(Citrus limonum)* is an uplifting oil that has a high energy vibration. It assists when you need to concentrate and focus, it enhances memory and clears the head. This oil also helps brighten those who suffer from depression or fearfulness. TOP NOTE

Marjoram *(Origanum marjorana)* is excellent for use in meditation and visualization because it brings greater clarity. This oil can be used to protect the home. Do not use in pregnancy. MIDDLE NOTE

Myrrh *(Commiphora myrrha)* has been used since ancient times in rituals, including meditation, where it enhances spirituality. It helps to lift depression and heal emotional issues. BASE NOTE

Orange *(Citrus vulgaris)* is an uplifting oil which dispels negativity and increases positive thinking. It brings a sense of joy and cheer, and helps us find peace. Use it in meditation to help build your confidence and to lessen anxiety and nervousness. TOP NOTE

Peppermint *(Mentha × piperita)* brings positivity and discourages negative thinking. It is stimulating, increases consciousness and clarity, and invokes healing energy during a visualization. It should not be used in pregnancy. MIDDLE NOTE

Rose *(Rosa centifolia, R. damascena, R. gallica)* is a nurturing oil which increases all aspects of love in our lives. It helps us to reach spiritual enlightenment, reduces tension, lifts depression and also encourages us to have more patience with others. BASE NOTE

Sandalwood *(Santalum album)* has been used traditionally in temples and for meditation. It is the best oil to use for meditation because it enhances spirituality. It soothes emotional volatility, reduces stress and eases insomnia. Being a spiritual oil, it creates harmony and peace. BASE NOTE

Ylang Ylang *(Cananga odorata)* helps to lift depression and promotes calmness and tranquility. This oil is an aphrodisiac and helps you let go of fears, anger and negative thoughts. It boosts self-confidence, increases feelings of love and is ideal to use for visualization meditations, as it strengthens your inner self. BASE NOTE

Although essential oils provide us with so many wonderful qualities on their own, blending several oils together tailors the scent to your specific needs.

It is good practice to blend oils with different notes (see *The calming basics*). For example, mix a top, middle and base note oil together to create a balanced and harmonious blend. By having each note represented, the blend will bring the most benefits without creating disharmony.

The following blends are for use in an oil burner. The blend can also be added to a bowl of steaming hot water placed close to where you are meditating.

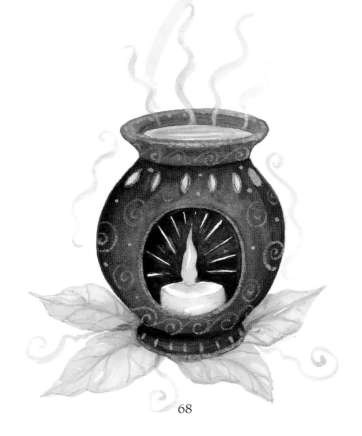

For lifting energy

2 drops each of basil, jasmine and lemon, or
2 drops each of orange and peppermint

To ease stress

2 drops each of bergamot, lavender and frankincense, or
2 drops each of rose and orange

To lift depression

2 drops each of bergamot, chamomile and myrrh, or
2 drops each of orange, lavender and ylang ylang

For higher meditative states

2 drops each of lemon, cinnamon and frankincense, or
2 drops each of basil, sandalwood and chamomile

To help concentration

2 drops each of lemon and peppermint, or
2 drops each of basil, lavender and jasmine

For boosting self-esteem and confidence

2 drops each of orange, fennel and ylang ylang

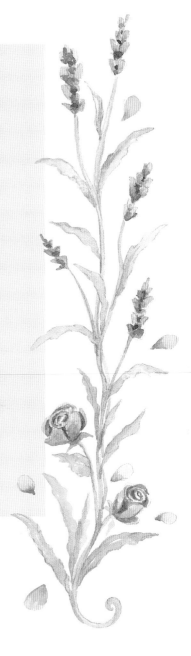

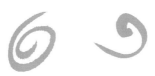

When using oils for meditation, choose one of the blends listed on p.69 or use a single oil that you feel will assist you. Alternatively, make up your own blends using the list of oils and their properties in *The calming basics* as a guide. Remember to try to have a mixture of top, middle and base note oils to make a balanced blend.

The following methods of use are all extremely simple, and the equipment you need can be as inexpensive as a single tissue.

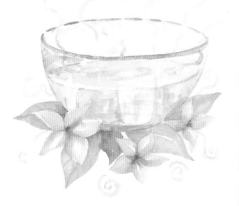

A good oil burner or diffuser will have a small bowl where water is heated slowly by a candle which sits beneath it. Add your chosen oil blend and the droplets of oil will vaporize with the mist from the heated water and fill your room with a delightful fragrance.

Paper Tissue

Place just a few drops of the essential oils onto a neatly folded tissue and tuck loosely into your clothing around your chest area to allow the oil vapors to drift upwards for you to inhale.

Bowl of Water

Place a small heatproof bowl close to your meditation space and use a heatproof mat to protect your furniture. Fill the bowl three-quarters full with boiling water from the kettle. Add your chosen blend of oils and then prepare yourself for meditation. The oils will vaporize in the steam and you will soon be enveloped in fragrant mist.

Cleaning your oil burner

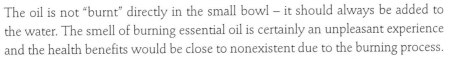

The best way to clean your oil burner is to add some methylated spirits to the bowl and wipe it out thoroughly with a paper towel. Ordinary detergent does not lift the sticky residue of the oils but it can be used to wash out the smell of methylated spirits from the bowl after the residue has been removed.

For electrical burners, put some methylated spirits onto a paper towel and wipe the plate thoroughly until all the residue has been removed.

The oil is not "burnt" directly in the small bowl – it should always be added to the water. The smell of burning essential oil is certainly an unpleasant experience and the health benefits would be close to nonexistent due to the burning process.

With this type of oil burner or diffuser, you have to remember to extinguish the candle after you have finished your meditation and also to top up the water bowl if you keep the candle lit for a extended period of time.

There are excellent candles on the market now which burn for up to eleven hours – perfect for the workplace, or for leisurely days at home on the weekends. Of course, you can extinguish the candle and relight it another time.

Electric oil burner/diffuser

This type of appliance creates a very low heat underneath the recessed plate where you place the oils. There is no need to add water to this type of burner as the temperature is so low that the oils are gently vaporized on their own without burning.

The advantage of this type of burner is that you can turn it on and literally leave it for several hours, except for the occasional replenishing of the oils. The disadvantage is that you don't have quite the same atmospheric "feel" that the candle-operated burners lend to a room. However, this type of burner is excellent for the workplace or any area where it is unsafe to have candles burning, such as the children's room.

Energy Awareness

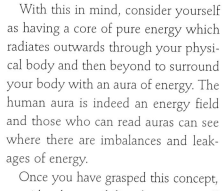

"We are energy or spiritual beings in physical bodies" is a statement often made by those people who recommend a daily practice of meditation, such as Dr Deepak Chopra and Dr Wayne Dyer (just two of many experts in the fields of psychology, mind/body connection work and quantum mechanics).

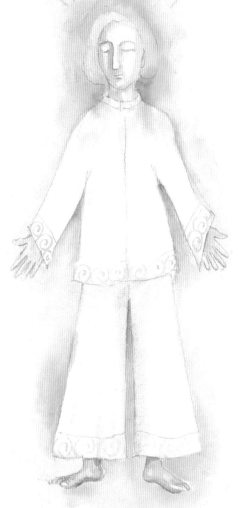

With this in mind, consider yourself as having a core of pure energy which radiates outwards through your physical body and then beyond to surround your body with an aura of energy. The human aura is indeed an energy field and those who can read auras can see where there are imbalances and leakages of energy.

Once you have grasped this concept, consider the possibility that we are all connected and come from the same universal energy. How else can you explain phenomena such as when the phone rings, the caller is the very person you have just thought about? Or when a person close to you says exactly what you were just thinking? Or when you are thinking about someone and then bump into them in an unusual place? These and many more situations occur in our lives regularly, and the theory is that we are connected by, and are part of, the very same energy.

To see a clear picture of yourself as a being of pure energy, imagine universal energy entering the crown of your head and flowing through all of your being – physical, mental, spiritual and emotional. Now see the way you give "energy" to others or to situations. For example, the simple flow of love between two people is a balanced energy "transaction". You both give and receive energy (love), and the relationship does not leave you depleted or overcharged with energy.

This is a simple picture of how the energy flows between us. Another example is when you are by the sea, in the bush or amongst nature of any kind. All of nature is alive with universal energy, and as we give and receive energy between ourselves, we also give energy to, and receive energy from, nature. This is why when we feel depleted of energy, we can sit beneath some trees in the park and simply rest. After a short time, we feel stronger, less vulnerable, and our inner strength becomes more apparent. Trees, plants and bodies of water provide us with pure energy. If you feel a little dubious, try sitting under, or close to, a tree next time you feel exhausted, and bring your awareness into your body and mind. After a short time, I guarantee you will feel different if your mind is aware.

In the following pages we look at how we lose energy, how we can avoid unnecessary loss and how we can recharge.

Using the energy principles mentioned so far, let us look at some situations that occur between people and how we lose energy.

Picture a married couple where the husband is very domineering and the wife is subservient and lacking in self-esteem. See them as beings of pure energy and imagine that much of the wife's energy is going to the husband while she tries to meet his demands and be what he expects her to be. She would feel constantly depleted, harangued and inadequate, and her sense of self would be close to nonexistent.

The husband, on the other hand, would be feeling quite strong from all this energy and may even make a point of commenting on his wife's so-called short-comings within earshot so that he could gain even more superiority (energy). His energy would be unbalanced, and to keep his supply coming in, excess he would have to be constantly making his wife feel small (depleted).

Now look at the person who is a real "drama queen", who sees every event as a problem or a real-life drama. See how they revel in their behavior and how they gain attention (energy) from other people's reactions and behavior during their "performances". Notice how drained you feel when you are around them.

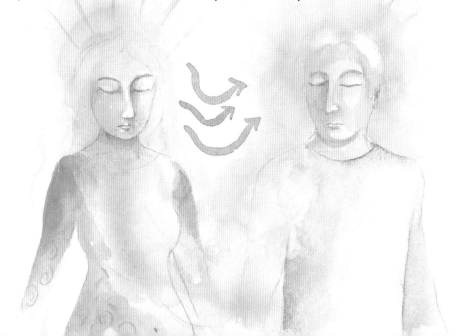

How do you feel when you have had an argument with someone? Do you feel energized or depleted? Does this depend on whether you won or lost the argument? Of course it does! If someone is constantly picking fights or arguments with others or enjoys harassing people to the point of a verbal or physical fight, their energy is very unbalanced. They feel small (depleted) and so to make themselves feel better on some level, however temporary, they may initiate a confrontation. The person may feel better (energized) afterwards, but this is temporary, and so they carry on finding ways to feel better or gain energy.

What happens when an abusive parent comments often on their child's inability to perform a task well? Do you think this helps the child to do better? What is happening energistically? The parent for some reason thinks their comments (a form of verbal abuse) will inspire the child to do better. Sure, it may work on some level but what is really happening is the child is losing self-esteem (energy) and the parent may perhaps feel a little righteous (energized). This may be an extreme case, consider subtle forms of this situation in your daily relationships with others. For example, a person may use sarcastic quips about their friends within earshot to get others to laugh. The laughter makes that person feel good (energized) but leaves the victims depleted.

Resentment of another person is actually a leakage of energy to the person who is being resented – explaining why one feels so tired when riddled with resentment. Anger directed at another is a way of gaining energy from that person, while acting aloof is a way of gaining attention (energy) from others. Talking nonstop to someone is a way of gaining energy and betrays an unbalanced state. Brooding and the use of "silent treatment" are ways of gaining attention (energy) from others who feel affected by this behavior. Tears and hysteria are also ways that of gaining another person's attention or energy.

While most of these behaviors are common everyday scenarios, it is very helpful for you to become more aware of how other people's behaviors affect your energy and vice versa.

To avoid your energy being lost unnecessarily, you first have to become aware of your own behavior with those you come into contact with on a daily basis.

Spend several days on the "observation platform", and watch how you interact with others. Keep a daily journal – as detailed or as brief as you like – highlighting when you have lost energy to, or gained energy from, another person. Also take note of when you feel genuinely good with someone – this will be when the energy flow is balanced and is flowing both ways. I have several friends whom I feel wonderful being around. In my mind I call our friendships "the mutual admiration society", because I know these friends love me unconditionally, as I love them. This is something I also experience with my family – we are fortunate enough to have loving and supportive relationships with each other.

When you compare the difficult relationships with the mutually satisfying ones, you can begin to see where the energy flow is out of balance. This is not to say you drop friendships or lovers because of this. However, it can help you pinpoint what behavior depletes your energy, and this gives you a chance to slowly change the mechanics of the friendship to bring about more harmonious interactions. This of course depends on how much the other person relies on the unbalanced interactions to gain energy or how honest you are being with yourself on the nature of the relationship. This contemplation can be quite confronting, but is beneficial if you are to reach a greater understanding of yourself.

Once you are armed with greater awareness of all the interplays of energy in your life, you can then choose which ones you want to avoid or step away from. For example, when another person is harassing you, observe the energy interplay with detached emotions – this allows you to choose simply not to become involved, so that you can retain your energy. However, if you have a friend who constantly depletes your energy, you may want to consider talking with them to try and change the nature of your relationship for the better.

Energy plus meditation

After doing the relaxation and white lighting exercises (see p. 21), sit quietly for a few minutes and focus on breathing slowly and deeply.

Picture yourself on the top of a hill, standing under a tree, overlooking a valley and other hills. Notice all the different shades of green in the grass and trees, and how blue the sky is. There are soft clouds drifting overhead and the sun is caressing your skin warmly. A gentle breeze is blowing and you notice the trees are swaying slightly.

Look at the energy pouring out of the trees and grass and picture it swirling around your body. Feel the energy pouring out of the tree you are standing beneath and look up into its magnificent branches. Stand with your back against the tree and feel its energy softly surround your body. As you stand quietly, you will notice that you cannot feel where your body ends and where the tree and air begin. You softly melt into the tree and become one with it. You can feel the energy course through your body, with the strength of the tree becoming your own. The wisdom of the ages found in this ancient tree pours into your being and you have memories of seasons coming and going for centuries – the ebb and flow of life is all around you.

Stand there, allowing the energies of the tree to pour through your being, bringing inner strength and compassion for all living things. Become immersed in endless time and nothingness for as long as you like.

Now slowly begin to feel the boundaries of your body and see yourself stepping out of the tree trunk. Picture your energy combining with that of the tree and imagine the beautiful flow of energy between you.

Slowly bring yourself back to the room, bringing with you feelings of peace and contentment. Wiggle your fingers and toes and become aware once more of your breath.

Energy interplay meditation

After doing the relaxation and white lighting exercises, sit quietly for a few minutes focussing on your breath.

See yourself interacting with someone close to you and see both of your energy fields or auras. Watch how the energy flows between you and how it sometimes travels more one way than another. Imagine that you have an argument and see how the energy travels more to the person who is the most indignant or angry. Now see yourself changing the interaction by choosing different behavior and different, kinder words in response to the anger and watch how the energy flow is altered. Notice how the energy flow can be altered by choosing different responses. Notice how the use of knee-jerk reactions makes the energy flow very unbalanced.

Now see yourself alone and imagine the universal energy pouring into the crown of your head and into your entire being. See your aura become full and vibrant.

Quietly return to your breathing and bring yourself back to the room gently.

RECHARGING AND CONSERVING ENERGY

Now that you begin to understand how energy works, learn how to recharge and conserve your energy by following some of the suggestions below.

Meditation

The simplest way to recharge your energy is through meditation. Daily or regular meditation practice will ensure that you remain centered, without the need to gain energy from others. You can follow the meditation exercise above from time to time or simply do the white lighting exercise each day to top up your energy and re-center yourself. Follow the exercises outlined in *Meditative techniques for every day* to ensure that you maintain centeredness as much as possible. This is how you can best ensure that your energy is as complete as possible and that you will be able to automatically relate to others in a healthy way.

Communing With Nature

As often as you can, visit a park, beach, forest, river, desert or any other place where you can commune with nature. Try to meditate in natural surroundings as often as you can, and picture the energy from the trees and water pouring into your being. Imagine your energy flowing back into nature in a continuous, replenishing flow.

A simple walk in the park can be just as beneficial and, if this is your only opportunity, walk there often, sometimes taking the time to rest under a tree.

Live With Awareness

Recognise power (energy) struggles with others and detach emotionally from those situations. Try to see others from their point of view and try to have compassion at all times. We are all doing the best we can, and while it may seem others could do much better, who are we to judge? Do not judge yourself or others, and promote harmony with all those with whom you come into contact. Do not become involved in gossip or backstabbing and keep your opinions to yourself. All this is negative behaviour which depletes your energy.

Personal Challenges

Live for now and take up those challenging hobbies you have always wanted to pursue. Recognize when fear is stopping you from undertaking challenges that will bring personal growth and satisfaction. Build your confidence and self-esteem by following pursuits which take you a little out of "your comfort zone". Do what you can to push past irrational fears so that you can truly "live" your life, not just simply exist.

Live With Thanks

Be mindful of the wonderful things in your life and give daily thanks to the universe for the blessings bestowed upon you – be it good health, the ability to work, a good job, or supportive family and friends.

Published by Lansdowne Publishing Pty Ltd
Sydney NSW 2000, Australia

Commissioned by Deborah Nixon
Text: Jan Purser
Designer: Sue Rawkins
Editor: Antonia Lomny
Cover illustration: Tina Wilson
Illustrator: Penny Lovelock
Production Manager: Kristy Nelson
Project Co-ordinator: Clare Wallis

National Library of Cataloguing-in-Publication Data
Castorina, Jan, 1960-.
  Meditation: easy techniques to help you focus and relax

  ISBN 1 86302 678 9.
  1. Meditation - Technique. 2. Relaxation. I. Title

  158.12

Set in Stempel Schneidler on Quark XPress
Printed in Singapore by Tien Wah Press (Pte) Ltd